# How I Healed My Teeth by Eating Sugar

## A Guide to Improving Dental Health Naturally

By Joey Lott

www.joeylotthealth.com

June 2014


Published by Archangel Ink

ISBN: 1500191280
ISBN-13: 978-1500191283

# Table of Contents

Preface 5

The Possibility of Healing Our Teeth 9

Dental Anatomy 14

Exploring Nutritional Building Blocks for Dental Health 19

Fat-Soluble Vitamins 22

Minerals 27

Demineralizing Substances 31

Protein 35

Metabolism 38

Diet 44

Supplements 59

Cleaning and Care 68

Remineralizing Paste 70

Oil Pulling 73

What Now? 76

Get My Future Books FREE 79

Connect With Me 80

One Small Favor 81

About the Author 83

# Preface

The title of this book is provocative. It is also true. I really did heal my teeth by eating sugar. Oh, and I did some other things as well, all of which I tell you in this book. When I say that I healed my teeth, I mean that I regrew dentin that filled in some fairly massive cavities. My teeth no longer hurt. They are strong and snug. And overall, they feel good.

The reason for the provocative title of the book is that I want to grab your attention and give you information that few are telling you. For one, I want you to know that healing your teeth is possible, because our teeth are alive. From a scientific standpoint, regrowth of some (though not all) of the tissues is entirely undisputed. Even more importantly, I want you to know that this healing doesn't necessitate rigid dietary protocols as others might have you believe - hence the suggestion that I healed my teeth by eating sugar.

This is a book about healing teeth naturally. That means that with the advice from this book, you may be able to regrow teeth (assuming the heart of the tooth is still in tact), reduce or eliminate cavities, firm up loose teeth, and improve gum health.

None of this is science fiction. Everything in this book is honest and real advice based on good science and anecdotal evidence that it can work.

There are other books on this subject, and there is also a good deal of information available for free on the internet on this subject. And much of it may work. However, my opinion is that much of that other information in books and on the internet is unnecessarily restrictive and complicated. While it may work for some people some of the time, in the long run, it may do more harm than help if one can actually stick with the rigid protocols. More likely, most people simply will not or cannot manage such a restrictive approach to their lives and health. So in this book I offer a much more manageable approach to natural dental health that is free of much of the dogma found elsewhere.

What you'll find in this book is that while I agree that some of the information that you will find elsewhere is solid (i.e. it certainly does seem that without adequate dietary minerals, including calcium, teeth cannot regenerate), I actually disagree with some of the foundational principles of much of both mainstream and alternative advice for tooth care. For example, nearly everyone claims that sugar is to blame for tooth decay. In fact, many, if not most, go so far as to suggest that starch too is to blame for tooth decay. Yet my experience runs contrary to this, and I also have found substantial evidence in my research that suggests that this common advice may well be misleading.

Apart from the contrary nature of this book, another thing that sets it apart is that this is the only book of which I am aware that shares about the incredible impact that metabolic health has on dental health. So while others suggest that you must eliminate all sugar and starch while guzzling cod liver oil in order to heal your teeth, in this book I present you with a different picture. In my research, metabolic health is key to dental health, and this means that above all you must eat enough. Eliminating foods from your diet is counterproductive.

If you're ready for a fresh, new perspective on natural dental healing that you can do yourself with an unrestrictive, enjoyable approach, then read on. You're in for a treat. I do not promise that you can get the same results as I did by applying the same principles, of course. However, I believe that the information in this book is some of the best on this subject.

# The Possibility of Healing Our Teeth

We've all had the experience of looking at our teeth and thinking to ourselves, "Oh, it's really too bad that I've let my mouth go so far into disrepair since now I'll be stuck with these pitted, weakened, loose, and sensitive teeth and receding gums for the rest of my life."

And yet, what very few of us know is that our teeth and gums can heal. Although we receive a popular message quite to the contrary, anecdotal evidence from thousands of people around the world suggests that under the right conditions it often is possible to restore health to our teeth and gums.

That has been my own experience, and I have heard others report similar results. Many people seem to feel that they must follow a strict dietary protocol to achieve these results, yet I do not believe that this is necessary. I do believe that it is important to eat lots of nutrient-dense foods to support dental health. However, I do not believe that it is necessary to restrict one's diet to extremes as many others suggest.

Here is my experience: I followed many strict and pure dietary regimens over the years, many of which involved greatly restricting or eliminating sugars and starches as many experts suggest one should do. Yet in reality. my dental health declined slowly over the years. Due to extreme anxiety and other emotional problems that I experienced (and have written about elsewhere), I ended up neglecting my teeth for years. Because of this, I formed many cavities. In fact, one cavity on one of my wisdom teeth was so big that I could stick the tip of my tongue into it.

My teeth became very sensitive to just about everything. They hurt, and they became loose in the sockets as well. Like many people,

I believed that what was done was done and there was nothing I could do about it.

However, when I put into practice the simple things that I outline in this book, I discovered that my teeth (and gums) began to heal. My teeth became less sensitive and firmed up in the sockets. My gums became healthier. They stopped bleeding and grew back up around the roots of the teeth from where they had receded. The cavities even began to fill back in. I didn't notice this until one day I tried to stick the tip of my tongue into that enormous cavity only to find that it had completely filled in with dentin!

In this book, I intend to share with you what I believe to be the easiest-to-follow guide on the subject of restoring health to teeth and gums through natural means. Unlike other books on this subject or information that you can find on the internet, the information in this book is relatively inexpensive, easy to do, and sustainable. Furthermore, this is a simple guide, presented in a direct fashion. There's not a lot of fluff or confusing and unnecessary scientific-sounding filler. The science contained within this book is straightforward, relevant, and easy-to-understand.

Whereas many protocols for tooth remineralization and natural dental health suggest restrictive diets and expensive supplements, I have found that little of that is necessary. In fact, many of the restrictive diets actually seem to hurt people's health in the long run, which then can lead to worsening dental health!

In this book, I will offer you honest information that is based on actual anecdotal experience as well as sound theory and research. Unlike other books, I see no need to make inflammatory claims against the dental industry or common dental practices. You are welcome to follow your dentist's suggestions if you wish. Nothing that I suggest in this book should be in conflict with your dentist's recommendations on a practical level, though your dentist may, of course, disagree with some of the claims that teeth can regrow. That is fine, though. Your dentist can disagree. You can follow the easy-to-do recommendations throughout the book, and you both can see what happens.

In other words, nothing in this book should be misconstrued as medical or dental advice, even though the subject of this book does deal with your health, including dental health. You are free to put into practice the ideas put forth in this book either independent of the advice of a dental professional or in conjunction with the advice of a dental professional. I have no desire to try and represent myself as a dental health expert. I'm just a normal person who happens to have researched these matters, tried a variety of extreme dietary protocols, and found some simple answers that have worked for me and for others. I hope that you find some benefit from what you read in this book as well.

# Dental Anatomy

Our bodies are living. Every part of them is alive. Just as your heart is alive, so too are your teeth alive. This may come as a surprise to you since we are often taught to think of our teeth as non-living structures, but when you look at the structure of teeth, you can see rather easily that they are, in fact, very much alive.

Now, to build a solid foundation of understanding, we're going to start by looking at the structure of teeth. This will be a little sciencey, but I'll keep it as simple as possible. So don't worry!

There are four major classifications of tissue that make up a tooth. Those are dental pulp, cementum, dentin, and enamel.

The dental pulp is a flesh-like tissue that connects the nerves and blood vessels from the rest of the body to the tooth. The pulp is at the core of the tooth, and the nerves and blood vessels pass through the roots of the teeth through the facial bones, and connect with the rest of the nervous and circulatory systems of the body. As long as the pulp is healthy, the rest of the tooth tissue can theoretically receive nutrition and other health-giving support from the rest of the body. Without the pulp, however, a tooth stands little to no chance of repairing itself.

The dentin tissue forms from the pulp, and it grows around the pulp. Dentin is composed primarily of mineral matter with a substantial amount of protein. Dentin is known to grow throughout the life of a tooth in response to various needs and stimuli. Dentin is thought to be necessary to support enamel.

Cementum is a mineralized tissue layer that forms around the dentin of the roots of a tooth. This tissue helps to connect a tooth to the socket. Specialized connective tissue called ligaments join the socket and the tooth by anchoring to the cementum.

Enamel is the hardest and most mineralized dental tissue. Enamel forms on the outer surface of the tooth above the gumline. Enamel is what allows us to chew relatively hard foods. Of course, due to the mineralized nature of enamel, it is also the most brittle type of dental tissue, as those of us who have chipped teeth can attest to. However, it is important to point out that while enamel has a high concentration of mineral content, it also contains some protein, which plays an important role in the living structure of enamel. So it is a mistake to think of enamel as a dead substance, because despite its hard structure, it is very much a living tissue.

The prevailing wisdom on the subject today seems to be that enamel does not regrow once it has been eroded. There have been some interesting studies in recent years that demonstrate the potential for stimulating enamel restoration, both through synthetic and natural means. So while most dentists will scoff at the suggestion that there is any potential to regrow enamel, some studies now show that it may not be so far-fetched.

While the debate continues as to whether one can actually regrow enamel under the right conditions, anecdotally, many people seem to benefit from providing adequate nutrition to support healthy tooth mineralization. At the very least, good nutrition can strengthen existing enamel, and it is at least theoretically possible that, under the right circumstances, it may be possible to repair enamel.

In a nutshell, as long as the dental pulp remains, it is theoretically possible to restore health to a tooth. Most seem to agree that healthy dental pulp combined with good nutrition and oral health care can regrow dentin and strengthen existing enamel. In many cases, this may be enough to vastly improve dental health. Though dentists have various opinions on the matter, many find that it is possible to improve dental health through natural means to the extent that it is possible to avoid fillings and even root canals in some cases. I am not suggesting that this will be your experience. It may or it may not.

However, anecdotally, many find this to be the case. Undoubtedly, at some point a dentist or two will write a scathing review of this book on the grounds that, in their opinion, it is reckless to suggest one might avoid a root canal. Yet again, anecdotally, many have reported good results with this approach for long periods of time. Ultimately, of course, the decision is yours - not mine, your dentist's, nor anyone else's.

# Exploring Nutritional Building Blocks for Dental Health

Many times, experts from both mainstream and alternative perspectives tend to focus on minerals for dental health. For example, we've all heard the claims that topical fluoride can strengthen teeth, and we've surely all heard the marketing hype about the importance of calcium for strong teeth.

While minerals certainly do seem to play a very important role in dental health, it is a huge mistake to think that minerals alone are the sole key to healthy teeth.

Hopefully, you can already see why this would be. In the preceding section we saw how dental pulp is essential for tooth health, and this type of tissue has a very low mineral content. Unlike dentin, cementum, or enamel, pulp is fleshy and contains large amounts of nerve and capillary networks. Because the pulp is essential for tooth health, simply adding more minerals overlooks the importance of this central tooth tissue. Pulp requires metabolic health, nerve health, and circulatory health and depends on overall health.

Furthermore, while 70% of dentin is mineral content, the remaining 30% is organic tissue and water, which includes proteins. So while minerals are undoubtedly important for the health of dentin, that is only part of the picture. Adequate nutrition and overall health is essential for dentin health.

Even the highly-mineralized cementum and enamel contain some proteins and other organic materials. The cementum connects to the socket by way of ligaments, which are composed of proteins, so proper nutrition and health are necessary to support these tissues.

Hopefully, you can begin to see that good dental health isn't as overly simplistic as popping a calcium supplement and applying topical fluoride.

In the following sections, we'll explore some of the specific ways in which various aspects of nutrition can play an important role in dental health.

# Fat-Soluble Vitamins

We've all heard of vitamins such as vitamin C or the B vitamin complex. Some of these vitamins are classified a water-soluble while others are classified as fat-soluble. While all vitamins may play an important role in dental health, the fat-soluble vitamins seem to play a particularly important role.

The fat-soluble vitamins include vitamins A, D, E, and K, and each of these vitamins is essential to overall health. Of these, A, D, and K seem to be the most important specifically for dental health.

Vitamin A is thought to be important for bone and tooth formation. Enamel contains some essential protein called keratin, which requires vitamin A for formation.

Typically, we are told that there are two types of vitamin A - carotenes (the orange and red pigments in vegetables such as carrots) and retinols (which are found only in animal foods). In reality, however, only retinols are true vitamin A. Theoretically, the human liver may be capable of converting carotenes into retinols, which is why carotenes are classified as vitamin A. However, not everyone converts carotenes well, so the only reliable sources of vitamin A are animal foods, of which liver seems to be the most potent source.

Vitamin D, which is more correctly classified as a hormone, is considered to be very important for bone and tooth health because it helps to move minerals into bone and teeth and out of tissues. This makes vitamin D doubly important for tooth health, because for a tooth to be healthy, both the non-mineralized parts (the pulp) and the mineralized parts need to be working well. If the pulp is mineralized, then it will not function properly. Vitamin D helps keep the pulp free of excess minerals while keeping the dentin, cementum, and enamel mineralized.

Many experts now claim that the majority of modern humans are deficient in vitamin D. Whether or not this is true, I cannot say. However, it is reasonable to understand how this might be so. Vitamin D is typically found in very small amounts in any food sources - animal and plant foods alike. Rather, the traditional source of vitamin D for humans is what the skin produces when exposed to sunlight. If naked humans living in tropical regions might be expected to form adequate vitamin D in this fashion, then it isn't hard to see how the average North American might be challenged in this regard.

Of course, humans have been clothed and living far away from the equator for a long time, so there must be traditional ways to increase vitamin D levels. It seems that sun exposure remains the tried and true means for increasing vitamin D levels, since adequate exposure during the warm months can theoretically raise levels sufficiently to carry one through the winter months. However, since most foods contain very small amounts of vitamin D, humans have also traditionally supplemented with high-vitamin specialty foods, such as cod liver oil, in regions where sunlight was a premium. (Don't worry, I'm not suggesting that you need to supplement with cod liver oil! We'll talk more about specific dietary and supplemental recommendations shortly.)

Finally, vitamin K is also thought to play an important role in tooth health. This vitamin is found to have a lot of important roles in human health, including a similar role to that of vitamin D in keeping minerals in teeth and bones while keeping them out of tissues. For this reason, vitamin K seems to be very important for keeping teeth strong and healthy.

Vitamin K is really a group of similar compounds, and within the category there are two distinct types, which are called K1 and K2. K2 is the form that is thought to be used within the human body. However, the body can convert some K1 into the more useable K2 form.

K1 is found in plant sources, including many leafy greens. However, K1 from plant foods generally has poor bioavailability, though the bioavailability can be more than doubled with the addition of dietary fat to the same meal.

K2 exists in animal foods as well as some specially-fermented foods in which bacteria produce K2. In fact, the food with the highest levels of K2 is natto, which is produced by bacterial fermentation of soy.

One last note regarding fat-soluble vitamins: since they are only soluble in fat, it is advisable to include adequate fat in one's diet. Without adequate dietary fat, it can be difficult for the body to properly metabolize the nutrients. What this means is that low fat diets (or diets with low amounts of saturated fat) tend to lead to deficiencies in fat-soluble vitamins, which can adversely affect dental health.

# Minerals

Although minerals are not the whole picture when it comes to dental health, they play an undeniably important role. Without adequate dietary minerals, it is all but impossible to enjoy good dental health.

When most people think of dental health, there are just two minerals that come to mind: fluoride and calcium. This oversimplification ends up being a detriment to many people's dental health, because dental health requires a lot more than just these two minerals.

To begin with, let me address fluoride. This is a very contentious issue, perhaps mostly due to the debate over water fluoridation. My personal preference is to avoid all supplemental fluoride. I live in a rural area with well water, and neither do I choose to use topical fluoride in toothpaste or otherwise. I personally do not feel that it makes sense for my own body. And, there is some good evidence that suggests that excessive fluoride exposure may have detrimental effects on the endocrine system, primarily impacting thyroid health, so I am glad to have no unnecessary fluoride exposure. My dental health has increased significantly in the years since I have moved from cities in which I had fluoridated water, so in my view, supplemental fluoride doesn't seem to be helpful.

However, frankly, it is such a contentious political issue that I don't see the merit in taking a strong stance for the purposes of this book as I suspect that would distract from its value. Rather, I believe that the issue of fluoride is one that each individual must make. If you feel that supplemental fluoride is important for your dental health, then continue what you are doing. If you feel that supplemental fluoride is harmful to your health, and you prefer to avoid it, then do so. Either way, I believe that the information in this book can be helpful to you, and I don't see that supplemental fluoride will greatly help or hinder.

With that out of the way, let's continue to look at the importance of minerals in terms of dental health.

Calcium certainly does seem to be an important mineral for tooth health. However, it is only one of the important minerals, and without the others in balance, calcium alone doesn't seem to be able to correct tooth problems. Furthermore, as indicated in the previous section, fat-soluble vitamins appear to be essential in terms of getting minerals, such as calcium, into teeth. So calcium without adequate fat-soluble vitamins doesn't seem to be very useful. In fact, without adequate fat-soluble vitamins, calcium and other minerals can end up in tissues, which can cause all sorts of health problems.

Weston A. Price was a dentist who is now famous (or infamous, depending on your view) for bringing to our attention the important role of nutrition in dental health. In his research there were significant differences in the diets of those who demonstrated good dental health versus those who demonstrate poor dental health. The two main differences that he found were between the levels of dietary fats and dietary minerals. In many cases, he found that those with good dental health ate approximately four times the minerals as those with poor dental health.

The minerals that are needed in the largest amounts are calcium, phosphorus, and magnesium. In addition, the body (and teeth) need all the trace minerals in smaller amounts. Of the trace minerals, those that are most significant for dental health include iron, copper, manganese, zinc, silica, and boron.

The good news is that as long as one eats enough quality, nutrient-dense food, then acquiring enough dietary minerals should not pose a problem. Neither does it need to require eating lots of "health" foods that no one enjoys eating. We'll take a look at this in more detail shortly.

# Demineralizing Substances

Many drugs, both prescription and illicit, interfere with proper mineralization within the body. Drugs such as antibiotics, anticonvulsants, steroids, diuretics, and acid blockers are examples of types of drugs that can interfere with mineral absorption, so if you are using any of these drugs, then you may need to factor in the effect that these drugs may be having.

Many foods include substances that interfere with mineral absorption as well. Some of the worst offenders are found in whole grains, legumes, and leafy green vegetables.

Whole grains, legumes, nuts, and seeds contain substances known as anti-nutrients such as phytic acid that can leach minerals from your body. Phytic acid is a bound form of phosphorus, which is an important mineral for health. However, because the phosphorus is bound, it is not available for your body to use. Moreover, phytic acid can further bind to other minerals, including phosphorus, calcium, magnesium, and so on, so it is best to minimize these anti-nutrients.

Most of the anti-nutrients in grains are found in the bran, so eating grain in which the bran has been removed can help in this regard. (We'll talk more about this in the Diet section.) Or, properly soaking and sprouting most grains and legumes will deactivate many of the anti-nutrients. (There are, however, some exceptions, such as brown rice, which lacks the enzymes to deactivate phytic acid.) Nuts and seeds are often difficult to properly sprout since most are heat-treated, which deactivates the enzymes that reduce anti-nutrients. Theoretically removing the skins of nuts or the hulls of seeds should reduce the anti-nutrient content, and roasting should reduce it even further. However, this is often impractical. In addition, nuts and seeds often have other unwanted substances, such as large amounts of polyunsaturated fat that goes rancid easily, so while nuts and seeds in moderation are fine, as with most things, it's probably not a great idea to gorge on them because you believe they are healthy. Rather, eat them if you genuinely crave them, and only in the amounts that you actually crave. In such cases they are probably good for you.

Oxalic acid is another common anti-nutrient found in a variety of foods. The fact is that many foods contain oxalic acid, and so it is impossible to avoid. However, many of the foods that people commonly eat large quantities of in an attempt to be healthy actually contain huge amounts of oxalic acid. Some examples of foods with extremely high levels of oxalic acid include kale, spinach, and chard. There's nothing wrong with eating these foods in moderation, of course, and if you genuinely enjoy eating large amounts of raw kale and spinach every day, then take that as a sign that they are good for you. However, the practice of eating massive servings of these foods every day strictly out of ideological reasons may be misguided as the oxalic acid may bind to minerals, depleting stores in the body. Taste and cravings are probably the best indicators. If you crave raw spinach, then eat it. If not, then cramming it down anyway may not be a great idea.

# Protein

As we saw earlier, all of the tissues of the teeth require some essential protein in order to remain healthy. Strangely, protein is often overlooked as an important part of dental health, and yet without adequate quality protein, it is unreasonable to expect your teeth to be healthy.

In fact, some websites even suggest that one should cut down on protein as a strategy to keep teeth healthy. This is a misguided recommendation, however. While excessive dietary protein to the extreme is sure to have negative health consequences, it seems very unlikely that anyone other than bodybuilders and others who force themselves to eat extreme amounts of protein is likely to have a problem of too much protein.

More likely, however, is that most people are not eating protein with a good balance of amino acids. More likely than not, many people are probably eating inflammatory proteins without a good balance of amino acids to nurture most of the body. The majority of the protein in the human body is collagen, and the teeth are no exception.

In fact, about 90% of the protein in dentin is composed of collagen, which is the same sort of protein that is found in abundance in bones, joints, eyes, and other organs, including the brain.

However, because most animal foods in the modern food system are deficient in collagen, you may not be getting enough of this important nutrient to support good health, including dental health. (We'll look at specific recommendations for how to remedy this in the Diet section.)

Also, although theoretically plant foods can supply a full array of amino acids, in practice this is very challenging for most people to achieve. Therefore, vegans may need to be especially careful in this regard. I was an ideological vegan for the better part of twenty years, and so I understand the ethical concerns of veganism, which are beyond the scope of this book to address. However, if your teeth aren't doing so great on a vegan diet, then there may be dietary issues undermining your dental health. These issues can include anti-nutrients, lack of fat-soluble vitamins, too little energy (calories), or poor quality or inadequate protein.

# Metabolism

Now that we've looked at the major building blocks for dental health, we're almost ready to take a look at some specific dietary recommendations. However, before we jump to that, there is one more very important factor that consider, and that is the role of metabolism in dental health.

I believe that metabolism is the big missing piece for many people's health. I am passionate about this subject because when I finally caught on to this, I turned around major health problems that had been plaguing me for years, including chronic fatigue, chronic Lyme disease, major insomnia, and some other problems that were negatively impacting my quality of life.

I also personally found metabolism to be a key component of improving my dental health, which is a connection I believe few people understand.

Metabolism simply refers to the energy system of your body, which involves everything from digestion to hormonal production to nerve impulses. Everything in the body is governed by how healthy the metabolism is.

While there are many possible factors that can determine metabolic health, one of the surest ways to harm metabolism is by chronically undereating.

Strange as it may seem, I find that many people nowadays are undernourished, even if they are eating a lot of volume. In fact, it seems that the healthier people try to eat, the greater the risk of under-nourishment. The reason is because a healthy metabolism requires a consistent input of food energy - also known as calories.

The truth is that to do proper justice to the subject of metabolism and the role that under-eating can play in harming metabolism would require another book. Necessarily, in this book I am going to leave a lot out of the discussion of metabolism. However, much of the necessary discussion for explaining this subject is only required because many of us are convinced that the only "healthy" diets are those that almost necessitate calorie restriction. As such, it often requires a great deal of convincing to explain to people that all the theories of healthy diets are meaningless unless a person is eating enough calories.

Truly, the facts are rather simple. While many of the diets that are promoted as ideal (such as whole foods, vegan, raw vegan, paleo, low carb, etc.) have convincing-sounding arguments, what most all of them leave out is that if one isn't getting enough energy from food (i.e. calories), then no amount of antioxidants or "life-force" or anything else will make up for that in terms of your basic needs. And in the face of a sustained calorie deficit, the body will slow metabolism.

Slowed metabolism has lots of symptoms associated with it, including:

- insomnia or disturbed sleep (often waking in the early morning with symptoms of high cortisol and/or adrenaline)

- depression
- anxiety
- food sensitivities or intolerances
- leaky gut
- irritable bowel
- edema or fluid retention
- intolerance to cold (and sometimes heat)
- cold hands and feet
- low or non-existent sex drive
- memory and/or cognitive problems
- dry skin, possibly rashes
- muscle and joint pain
- falling hair
- weight gain or weight loss (weight gain is more typical, but weight loss can result, particularly in chronic hypometabolic cases when a person has difficulty consuming enough food)
- frequent urination - particularly at night
- fatigue

If you experience any of those symptoms and/or your temperature is consistently less than 98.6 degrees Fahrenheit (37 degrees

Celsius) or your resting pulse is under 65 beats per minute, then you likely have a slowed metabolism.

A slowed metabolism means that your whole body's health will be compromised, including dental health. Remember that dental health isn't just about minerals. It also involves living tissue that is connected with the rest of the body. If your metabolism is slowed and therefore your body isn't functioning optimally, then that will make it very difficult for your teeth to be healthy.

If you are eating too little, then it will be all but impossible to improve your metabolism.

When I first learned of how much healthy weight-stable people eat, I was shocked. I had been accustomed to eating far less than that. And it also easily explained why I felt so terrible.

When healthy, weight-stable people are studied to find out how much they actually eat (versus how much they report), it turns out that pregnant and lactating women of all ages, as well as men under the age of 25, eat 3500 calories a day. Men aged 25 and over, as well as women under the age of 25, eat 3000 calories a day. And women who are neither pregnant nor lactating and who are aged 25 or over eat 2500 calories a day.

So, if you have a slowed metabolism and you are eating less than those figures suggest and you aren't feeling so great, then you might want to consider eating more. There are no guarantees, of course. However, anecdotally, I'm far from the only one who has experienced health benefits from eating more, and those health benefits have included improvements in dental health.

I do understand that you may have reservations about eating more. Most people do, especially because most people seem to be convinced that they are too fat. Yet I encourage you to set aside what you think you know about these things, and instead ask your body what you need. If your body needs more energy, then you might consider that your ideological diets have not been helping you.

# Diet

Almost all of the popular advice for how to improve dental health through nutrition ends up being unnecessarily restrictive, in my opinion. It seems that almost universally everyone who offers nutritional advice for dental health demonizes sugar, and then many of the advocates of traditional diets (such as the Weston A. Price Foundation) suggest that even many natural sugars are problematic. Many will even go so far as to recommend that one eliminates carbohydrates (except fiber, of course) entirely!

In my own experience this is not only unnecessary, but it can sometimes be harmful. This is why the diet that I recommend is much more lenient than most of what you'll find elsewhere.

I *do* believe that it is sensible and wise to stick to real foods that are as nutrient-dense as possible - within reason. And, there are some important caveats, as we'll explore together. So I'm not suggesting that it is necessarily advisable to eat a diet consisting of nothing more than Twinkies, Lifesavers, and chocolate chip cookies, but neither does it seem advisable to me to swing to the extreme of eliminating all sugar and all refined starches and only ever eating cod liver oil, high vitamin butter oil, and kale, as it would seem some suggest.

I believe there is a sensible, practical, and sustainable middle ground. This involves what I call "intuitive eating" coupled with an awareness of eating enough to support metabolic health and some suggestions for foods to try to include regularly. This doesn't have to be a rigid diet. In fact, it is best if it is not(!), because a rigid diet isn't usually sustainable.

Furthermore, my suggestions are actually in line with some of the findings that Dr.

Price reported in his book, *Nutrition and Physical Degeneration.* In that book, he reported that he recorded improvements in dental health of children who received a single supplementary meal daily in which they ate cod liver oil and high-vitamin butter oil along with a quality meat broth. Even though these children were otherwise still eating the same diets that had led to tooth decay (which reportedly consisted largely of refined grains and sugars), this simple supplementation resulted in dental health improvements.

So it does not seem to me that it is necessary or even desirable to radically change one's diet in a restrictive fashion as many modern health proponents suggest we should. My observation is that many, if not most, people who do so end up with worse health problems than when they started the restrictive diet. This may take months or it may take years. However, I see it happen time and time again. I believe there is a better way.

The following are my recommendations for a better way.

There are three basic guidelines to the diet that I recommend:

1. One must eat enough (see guidelines for adequate daily calories from previous section) from a variety of foods, including all macronutrients (fat, protein, and carbohydrates).
2. One must eat enough nutrient-dense foods to supply adequate vitamins and minerals.
3. One must reduce toxins and anti-nutrients to a sustainable minimum.

In practice, this is pretty easy to do. Or, I should say, it is theoretically easy to do, and once one gets the hang of it, it is very easy to do. However, the biggest challenge that most people have is that they refuse to comply with the first guideline because they are adhering to a restrictive diet because of ideology. That is typically the biggest hurdle.

Here is where I tell you again that my dental health improved dramatically when I started eating massive amounts of sugar.

Why would that be so? How is it that sugar could help my dental health? I don't know, but I suspect it has a lot to do with metabolism. Eating a lot of sugar helped me to fuel a healthy metabolism. Until that happens, it is darn near impossible to sustain good health, including dental health. Does that mean that there aren't people who live off of a 1200 calorie a day diet with absolutely no sugar and have stellar dental health? Of course not. There probably are some people who manage that, but I wasn't one of them. And you probably aren't either.

My experience and the experiences of many others I have communicated with on this subject is that it is very difficult (as in, almost impossible) to eat enough to fuel a healthy metabolism *and* stick to a "perfect" and "healthy" diet, such as raw vegan or low carb paleo. That doesn't mean that it is strictly impossible, of course. Some people can do it, but most of us cannot. So my finding is that eating *enough* is more important than eating only the "right" foods.

Once you're eating enough, you can start to try to eat enough while only eating the "right" foods if that still feels important to you, but in my experience, getting the metabolism functioning is the most important first step.

I personally got my metabolism up by eating massive amounts of easy-to-digest energy sources, including lots of whole dairy, butter, sugar, white rice, potatoes, and fruit juice. Of course, apart from the milk and butter, these foods are usually what the "experts" tell us are the worst for dental health. Yet, I found exactly the opposite, and I'm not alone.

Really, I believe that a lot of well-intentioned people today are placing unnecessary restrictions on their diets and suggesting that others do the same simply because they are basing their advice on ideologies that they never actually tested themselves. Dr. Price found that adding in nutrient-dense superfoods was sufficient to improve dental health in children. He didn't report that the children had to eliminate all grain and all sugar. And this is consistent with my own experience. In fact, my dental health deteriorated during the times when I eliminated all grain and all sugar, and it improved when I added grain and sugar back into my diet. I believe this is largely because of metabolic health and not because of the particular foods.

Others may find that their dental health improves when they remove all sugar from their diet, but this may be coincidental. The elimination of sugar may not have caused the improvement in dental health. It may have been other factors, such as including more nutrient-dense foods or more fat-soluble vitamins.

In practice, I find that *enough* food is far more important than the ideologically correct food.

The second guideline is to eat enough nutrient-dense food to supply the necessary vitamins and minerals to improve dental health. This seems to be just as important as the first guideline.

In practice, it seems that the most important foods are quality fats and high-mineral foods. Some of the real superstar foods here include the following:

- Butter
- Coconut oil
- Saturated animal fat

- Whole milk
- Collagen-rich foods
- Mineral-rich broths (such as bone broths)
- Egg yolks
- Organ meats - particularly liver from grass-fed ruminants
- Mineral-rich salt

Although I like to be provocative with my claim that I improved my dental health by eating massive amounts of sugar, truth be told, I was mostly eating organic, cane sugar with the natural molasses still in tact. This form of sugar contains not only large amounts of energy, but also a lot of minerals and vitamins. I am certainly not suggesting that refined sugar should be demonized because I ate a fair amount of refined cane sugar as well. However, I suspect that for dental health, sugar with a higher mineral content is probably preferable to sugar that is further refined. So most of the sugar that I eat conforms to all three of the guidelines given here.

In addition to eating sugar, I also eat lots of nutrient-dense foods. I drink lots of whole milk (I have a preference for raw milk when possible, though I'm not convinced that it is necessary that milk be raw as many people claim). I eat lots of butter. I eat lots of egg yolks. I eat a lot of gelatin. And I believe that these foods really do improve dental health.

Some people claim that they have intolerances to dairy. Anecdotally, however, dairy - especially whole milk - does tend to be very useful for improving dental health. It contains a lot of minerals that are hard to find from food unless one is eating a lot of bone broth. It also contains valuable quality fats, so it's worth making a few notes on this subject.

To begin with, very few people are genuinely intolerant of dairy. You may be one of those people. Most people are not, even though they think they are. Rather, many people find that if they aren't genetically unable to digest milk well, then they are able to eat dairy when they do two things. First, improving metabolism often makes a big improvement in all food intolerances. Secondly, actually eating dairy on a regular basis tends to improve things. Furthermore, some people tolerate unhomogenized milk better than homogenized. It is now possible to find unhomogenized milk in many natural food stores. And others find that raw milk is easier to digest than pasteurized milk. While I do personally have a preference for raw milk, I am able to digest pasteurized, unhomogenized milk just fine.

For those who do not want to or cannot eat dairy, then bone broth is the next best thing. In fact, bone broth is a wonderful food in many respects. The only downside to bone broth is the amount of work involved. (Gelatin, which I mention in the next section, is a convenient way to get the collagen benefits of bone broth without having to make bone broth. However, gelatin does *not* have the mineral benefits of bone broth. So for those who cannot or will not eat milk nor bone broth, then supplementing with something such as calcium bentonite clay, as mentioned later in the book, may be the next best option.)

While many "experts" claim that one should eat *only* nutrient-dense whole foods, I don't believe this is necessary or even necessarily helpful. As I indicated earlier, Dr. Price reported that simply *adding* nutrient-dense foods to existing diets of some populations resulted in improvement in dental health. This is consistent with my own findings, so I caution against becoming fanatical about eating *only* nutrient-dense whole foods, because in practice it can backfire and work against you.

The third guideline is to reduce toxins and anti-nutrients to a minimum. This is important because many toxins and anti-nutrients will disrupt health in a variety of ways, which can lead to dental health problems.

A lot of toxins, such as pesticides, chemical food additives, and various chemicals in cosmetics, are known to be endocrine disruptors, which means that they interfere with hormonal balance. This can cause harm to overall health, including mineral balances, so keeping these toxins to a minimum is a good precaution.

When possible, it is ideal to eat food grown or raised without chemical pesticides or fertilizers and without added drugs, as are often added to conventionally-raised animals since the drugs can cause hormonal problems as well as mineral imbalances. When buying packaged foods, look for those without any chemical additives.

Anti-nutrients, as we've already discussed, are substances in foods that can leach nutrients from your body. I find that it is best to minimize unsprouted whole grains, legumes, nuts, and seeds in the diet, for example, and it seems to be best to eat small amounts of a variety of vegetables, rotating them over time to minimize the anti-nutrients in any one of them. This is why I personally believe that the current green smoothie and green juice fads may be misguided. Certainly there isn't likely to be anything wrong with eating leafy green vegetables on occasion. However, eating large amounts of the same green vegetables every day, year round may be a mistake. It seems unlikely that any traditional cultures would have done this since they would have eaten in season out of necessity. Eating moderate amounts of a variety of different vegetables (that you actually enjoy) is a good idea, of course. I am just suggesting that force-feeding yourself massive amounts of kale and chard in an attempt to be healthy may be misguided.

Although this practice of reducing anti-nutrients may result in sometimes eating refined carbohydrates, I don't see this as a big problem. While it may be problematic to eat refined grains as the staple food (simply because refined grains don't offer a lot of vitamins and minerals), I don't believe it is actually a problem to eat refined grains in moderation. In fact, I have personally found benefit from it. Refined grains are essentially pure starch, which is pure energy (though they do have some protein and a small amount of fat as well). While refined grains are stripped of much of the micronutrient content, this is not likely to be a problem when the diet includes nutrient-dense foods. And, in fact, it seems that refined grains are much better than unsprouted whole grains, because they are free of the anti-nutrient problem.

Many people want to be purists and eat only sprouted whole grains (since sprouting reduces the anti-nutrient content of grains, beans, nuts, and seeds). This is fine, of course. However, many people end up with a calorie deficit when they do this, so if you have a slowed metabolism, then I encourage you to consider focusing on improving metabolic health *first* before trying to be a purist.

The other anti-nutrient that is worth mentioning here is polyunsaturated oils such as canola, soy, corn, and safflower. While small amounts of polyunsaturated fat seems to be fine, large amounts work as a metabolism suppressant. Saturated fat, on the other hand, appears to have a beneficial effect on metabolism, so it would seem that, in terms of metabolic health as well as dental health, one would be best off to minimize polyunsaturated fat (within reason) and maximize saturated fat (within reason).

Overall, hopefully you can begin to see how these three guidelines work together to outline a diet that can be inclusive, enjoyable, sustainable, and healthy. Very little in this diet is excluded. In fact, nothing is strictly excluded. Rather, the first and most important guideline is that you must eat enough. Then, I suggest that you include some foods that most people find to be delicious and enjoyable. For example, butter and collagen-rich broth tend to improve the flavor of most foods. And then finally, there are just a few ideas for ways to minimize unnecessary toxins and anti-nutrients so as to maintain hormonal and mineral balance. It is not advisable to be neurotic or fanatical about any of this. In fact, trying to be a purist just produces stress, which undermines health. I honestly believe it is best to enjoy a stress-free diet that includes lots of delicious and palatable foods while simply ensuring that you are *also* eating some nutrient-dense foods, such as those listed previously. Let your appetite be your guide. Eat delicious food. Enjoy what you eat. Have no restrictions based on ideology, which means you shouldn't restrict foods based on anything in this book, either. Rather, just *don't force* yourself to eat or to restrict anything because you think it is healthy.

# Supplements

The idealists among us may want to achieve perfect health without any supplements whatsoever. This is fine except that it usually doesn't work. I find that some good quality supplements are really helpful in this regard.

However, unlike many of the self-proclaimed experts who write on this subject of natural dental health, I do not personally believe that it is necessary or even helpful to rely on super expensive and "pure" supplements.

Dr. Price studied the effects of supplementing diets with cod liver oil as well as high-vitamin butter oil, which is made by centrifuging the spring butter from grass-fed cows. He found very favorable results with these two supplements. As a result, most "experts" now recommend that people supplement with cod liver oil and high-vitamin butter oil.

There are a few problems with this, however. For one thing, these two supplements are very expensive. And for another thing, they don't always work for people. In fact, some people react badly to cod liver oil.

Dr. Price himself warned of the negative health effects of poor quality cod liver oil, and there is good reason to believe that most, if not all, cod liver oil on the market would fit the definition of poor quality cod liver oil given by Dr. Price. While the fermented cod liver oil (currently only produced by Green Pasture) does seem to be better tolerated by most when compared to other cod liver oil products, I'm not convinced that it is worth the price. And still, some people react badly to it.

So, while I have no desire to dissuade you from purchasing fermented cod liver oil and high-vitamin butter oil if you wish to do so, I do wish to make it known that I do not believe that they are necessary.

While it is usually a mistake to try and reduce a food to vitamin or mineral components, nonetheless, I suspect that much of the benefit of these supplemental foods is due to the fat-soluble vitamin content. As such, I believe that it is possible to obtain the same benefits (if not greater benefit) at less cost and with greater ease with a few simple and inexpensive supplements combined with real, nutrient-dense food.

I have personally gotten really wonderful results from a daily vitamin D/K combination liquid supplement. I have found that the Thorne liquid D/K combination works really well for me. (I have no affiliation with Thorne.) There are likely other good quality liquid D and K products. I can only recommend Thorne because that is the one that I have personally found to be useful.

When you are looking for D and K, I recommend a liquid in oil that is not soy oil. Good oil bases are usually olive oil or medium chain triglycerides, which is derived from coconut or palm oil. Also, look for products that have limited or no additional ingredients. The Thorne product I use has added tocopherols, which are vitamin E added presumably as an antioxidant. Some products contain weird chemical additives, and I would steer clear of them since I don't know what those additives do.

Most literature that I have read on vitamin D suggests that D3 is the preferable form (though many say it makes no difference whether it is D2 or D3), and it is safe to take at least 4000 IU daily. There is a lot of scary advice to avoid taking "too much" vitamin D because of the potential for overdose. However, upon actually examining this, it turns out that overdose seems to be difficult to achieve. I have read of some accidental overdoses in which people were unknowingly taking over 200,000 IU a day for months (because of a manufacturer error) before noticing symptoms. Discontinuing supplementation resolved those problems from what I have read. Standard recommendations range from 2000 IU to 4000 IU a day, and these seem to be safe. I'm no expert on the matter. However, I've read quite a lot on the subject, and if you want to be conservative, then 2000 IU to 4000 IU seems to be the right range for daily supplementation. And since vitamin D is fat-soluble, you can also take larger amounts less frequently, if you prefer. For example, you could take 14,000 IU once a week, which would be the equivalent of 2000 IU daily.

From what I have read about vitamin K, the recommendations are all over the place. However, it does seem reasonable to supplement with K2 (versus K1) since it would seem to be the form that the body prefers. The reports that I have read so far suggest that there is no actual upper limit with vitamin K. It doesn't seem to be toxic, even in very large doses. I don't see the sense in being extreme, though. I have actually taken large doses (15 mg daily) without noticing any particular benefit. And so for the money, I prefer to just take the Thorne D/K liquid, which supplies 200 mcg per 1000 IU of D. Therefore, if I take 2000 IU of D, then I take 400 mcg of K. This works just as well for me as taking the large amounts of K.

In addition to the D/K supplement, I eat lots of butter. Although it is doubtful that pasteurized butter contains much vitamin K and some of the other purported benefits of high-vitamin butter oil, it seems to work well enough for me, and it is just a tiny fraction of the cost.

Many people claim that eating liver is important for health. Personally, I actually very much like liver. I find it to be delicious. And yet, I don't eat a lot of it. So while I have little doubt that liver is a wonderful and nutritious food, I don't believe that it is as essential as some would have you believe. Of course, this is all relative. As I have already said, I eat a lot of butter and whole dairy, so I likely get a good amount of fat-soluble nutrients in that way. If I didn't eat so much butter, then perhaps liver would be more important.

Another supplemental food that I really like, and one that I believe has helped me tremendously, is gelatin. Gelatin is a protein produced from collagen, and so gelatin is a really convenient way to eat more of this really important and nourishing protein. I have read that adding gelatin to other protein-containing foods makes the protein more digestible. Certainly it feels that way. And as I have stated previously, collagen is the most abundant protein in the human body, including in the teeth, so eating gelatin is a really simple and easy way to provide this important nutrient.

Since collagen is the most abundant protein in most animals, then the traditional practice of eating the entire animal ensured adequate dietary collagen. However, in the modern food system, most of us have little access to the collagen-rich parts of the animal. While we usually can find bones to make into collagen-rich bone broth, this takes a lot of time that many of us simply don't have, so gelatin is a convenient alternative.

I purchase beef gelatin from a company called Great Lakes. A natural food store in my area carries it, but if you cannot find it locally in your area, you can find it on the internet. In fact, there is currently a vendor selling it on Amazon.com for less than the local natural foods store's price, so you can find it at very reasonable prices online if you look.

I have just one more supplement to recommend to you, which is calcium bentonite clay. I credit this clay as being the single most effective thing I have done for my dental health. Of course, I know that it's never just one thing. It's all of the things together - the butter and the gelatin and supporting a healthy metabolism all included. Yet I personally feel that adding supplemental clay has made a huge difference in my dental health.

I have used a variety of clays, and at present I believe the best is a calcium bentonite clay from a company called Earth's Living Clay (www.earthslivingclay.com). I have no affiliation with the company, and I presently make no commission from any sales based on my recommendation. However, after trying lots of clays, I feel that the clay they sell is very high quality and very affordable.

I sprinkle a small amount of clay into my drinks every day, and I notice a difference. Furthermore, I also use the very same clay to brush my teeth (more on that later), and I find that that makes a big difference as well.

In summary, I honestly believe that a few inexpensive supplements can make a big difference. Whereas many people recommend cod liver oil and high-vitamin butter oil that will run you up to $100 per month, I personally find that I get better results from less expensive supplements.

The Thorne D/K liquid can last for many months and works out to just pennies a day. The gelatin too can last for months depending on how much you use, and so it is very inexpensive. Likewise with the clay. I purchase a one pound bag of clay for $16 several months ago, and I am still using it.

# Cleaning and Care

I was sick for many years. Very sick. I had chronic Lyme disease, and for several years I could barely even stand up. So I let my tooth cleaning practices go by the wayside. I literally did not brush my teeth for several years.

I tell you this to put things in perspective. I'm not suggesting that it is preferable not to brush your teeth, because I don't feel that way. Now that I can, I do brush my teeth, and I'm glad for it. However, I point this out because many of us have been led to believe that we must brush and floss fanatically or else all our teeth will fall out. The truth seems to be somewhere between these extremes.

As I have already said, I now prefer to brush my teeth rather than not. And, I also enjoy flossing my teeth on occasion. However, I now suspect that brushing and flossing multiple times every day may be detrimental. I think there's a balance to find.

# Remineralizing Paste

What I find, and what many other also report, is that brushing and/or rinsing with a "remineralizing paste" is far more effective than using a conventional toothpaste, both in terms of cleaning and improving tooth strength. In fact, many conventional toothpastes include ingredients (such as glycerin) that can interfere with tooth health, so many people find that ditching the conventional toothpastes is a great benefit to their dental health.

Many people have their own preferences for remineralizing paste ingredients.

Personally, I like to brush with plain calcium bentonite clay. I find that it leaves my teeth feeling clean, fresh, and healthy.

Other people like to use other ingredients. Some of the most popular ingredients include: baking soda, sea salt, diatomaceous earth, powdered egg shells, coconut oil, and xylitol. Each of these ingredients has potential benefits. Some, such as baking soda and salt, can potentially be irritating to gums over the long run, though plenty of people have been brushing with these ingredients without problems for decades.

Although I personally enjoy brushing with just a small amount of clay, this practice isn't for everybody. Many people are accustomed to using toothpaste, and so they prefer to continue to use something similar. As I have mentioned, conventional toothpastes, even many "natural" toothpastes, include ingredients that may not be good for teeth, including glycerin and things such as sodium lauryl sulfate. So for those who are serious about remineralizing their teeth, it would seem to be best to avoid conventional toothpaste.

You can, of course, make your own "toothpaste" by combining some of the ingredients that I have listed earlier. Many people find that mixing some clay with coconut oil to form a paste is a nice way to do this. And then, because many people enjoy flavored toothpastes, they will add natural 100% pure essential oils (do not use synthetic fragrance oils for this purpose) to the toothpaste.

Of course, you may not want to do this yourself. In that case, should you want to get the benefits of a natural, remineralizing toothpaste without having to do it yourself, then you can purchase pre-made products. There are several remineralizing toothpaste products on etsy, for example. In fact, my partner Sarah makes remineralizing toothpaste, which she sells here on her etsy shop:

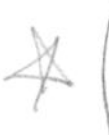
http://www.etsy.com/shop/EarthMamaMagicHerbs

# Oil Pulling

Oil pulling is another popular technique for mouth care. I have never done this practice daily, though I have experimented with it off and on over the years since I first heard of it back in 2005.

I find it to be a really nice practice that leaves my mouth feeling really clean. Frankly, if I could get into the practice of it, I feel that it would be very good for my mouth. The thing that holds me back from that is simply convenience; it is not the most convenient practice in the world.

Oil pulling is said to be a traditional Ayurvedic practice going back thousands of years. I can neither confirm nor deny this, though it does seem to be a reasonable claim.

It is said that the traditional practice of oil pulling uses sesame seed oil.

I do not believe that it matters what oil one uses, so long as it is a food-safe, non-toxic oil. And it may be that an oil such as coconut oil that has added antibacterial properties may be preferable to sesame oil.

I believe that even plain water is probably adequate for the practice. I am not convinced that there is necessarily anything special about oil that makes it better for this practice when compared to water. Oil is nice, however. So when I do oil pulling, I personally like to use coconut oil.

The practice is very simple. All you need to do is place a small amount of the oil (or water) in your mouth and begin to swish it around. Continue to swish it around for as long as you can stand. Many "experts" suggest that 20 minutes is the ideal. (Now you can understand, perhaps, the inconvenience factor.)

As you swish the oil or water in your mouth, you should be sure to swish it between your teeth and around the space between your gums and your lips. The idea is to thoroughly clean your mouth by massaging it with the swishing oil or water. This is a deep cleaning - far more thorough than simply flossing or brushing alone.

Some of the claims for oil pulling are a bit of a stretch, in my opinion. I don't think there is any need to make fantastical claims. It is enough that the practice gives your mouth a thorough cleansing, and if other benefits happen to come along with it, then that is wonderful.

If you feel so inclined, then consider giving oil pulling a try. Many people swear by it. I find it to be quite nice, though I have yet to get in the habit of doing it daily. I find that even once in a while is beneficial. It doesn't necessarily have to be every day. A once a week deep clean is quite lovely.

# What Now?

So there you have it - a simple, practical way in which to begin to improve dental health. This information, when put into practice, often helps people to regrow dentin, fill in cavities, improve tooth mineralization, firm up loose teeth, improve receding gums, and more.

Of course, none of this happens magically. You have to actually do it. However, hopefully, I have presented you with a system that is simple to do and easy to maintain. None of this should be particularly restrictive or unpleasant.

So how can you best get started? Well, here's a summary of my recommendations:

First off, understand that your teeth are alive, and as such, they can heal when you support them properly. The most important thing you can do to support your teeth is to provide your body with enough energy to fuel a healthy metabolism. So if your metabolism is slow, then fuel it with metabolism-boosting food, and lots of it.

Next, without restricting your diet, make sure to add in lots of nutrient-dense foods. Be especially liberal with quality fats such as butter, coconut oil, and saturated animal fats. Eat lots of quality, mineral-rich food, and eat enough quality protein to support growth in your body. Eat foods that you enjoy eating, and add a little extra butter or quality broth because these foods not only make everything taste better, they add important nutrients to your diet.

Then consider supplementing with a quality vitamin D/K liquid and a small amount of calcium bentonite clay. These two supplements along with gelatin seem to be among the best for improving dental health.

Lastly, ditch harsh toothpastes, and clean your teeth using natural remineralizing products. Oil pulling is a great way to get a deep clean and nourish your mouth, though not apparently essential in every case.

My belief is that all of this is possible to do inexpensively and enjoyably. I sincerely hope that you discover vibrant health, including dental health.

# Get My Future Books FREE

If you enjoyed this book (Hey, if you made it this far it couldn't have been that bad), you'll probably enjoy many of my other books about health and wellness. And you can get all my new releases in health and wellness for free by signing up for my mailing list at www.joeylotthealth.com. It's simple, it's free, and it's totally honest and legitimate. Nothing scammy or spammy or anything else like that (i.e. I won't be trying to sell you The 7 Dirty Underground Top Secret Weird Tricks for Rock Hard Abs or Young Living Oils). It's just about free books for those who appreciate my work, because I appreciate YOU. Simple as that.

# Connect With Me

I welcome your questions, comments, and feedback of any kind. Please feel free to email me at joeylott@gmail.com. I am now receiving so many emails that I cannot always reply to every email. I do read them all, and I do my best to reply to as many as possible. For the benefit of others, I may choose to publish my response to your email on my blog or in book format. I will maintain your privacy and anonymity if I choose to publish my response.

# One Small Favor

My sincere goal in writing is to share something that may be of value to you. And I endeavor to do so while keeping the costs low for readers. The success of my books and my ability to reach other readers who may benefit from my books depends in large part on having lots of thoughtful, honest reviews written about my work. You would do me a great favor if you would please take a moment to generously write a review of this book at Amazon.com. This will only take a few minutes of your time, and you will be helping me a great deal. I sure would appreciate it.

# About the Author

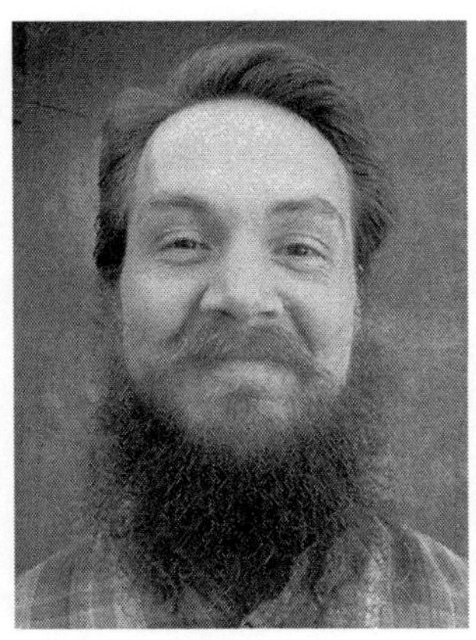

"The secret to happiness is to let go of everything - see through every assumption."

Beginning at a young age Joey Lott experienced intensifying anxiety. For several decades he lived with restrictive eating disorders, obsessions, compulsions, and an inescapable fear. By the time he was 30 years old he was physically sick, emotionally volatile, and mentally obsessed with keeping any and all unwanted thoughts and experiences at bay.

At this time Lott was living on a futon mattress in a tiny cabin in the woods. He was so sick that he could barely move. He was deeply depressed and hopeless. All this despite doing all the "right" things such as years of meditation, yoga, various "perfect" diets, clean air, and pure water.

Just when things were at their most dire, a crack appeared in the conceptual world that had formerly been mistaken for reality. By peering into this crack and underneath all the assumptions that had been unquestioned up to that moment, Lott began a great undoing. The revelation of this undoing is that reality is utterly simple, ever-present, seamless, and indivisible.

Lott's books provide a glimpse into the seamless, simple, and joyous nature of reality, offering a glimpse through the crack in conceptual worlds. Whether writing about the ultimate non-dual nature of reality, eating disorders, stress, disease, or any other subject, he offers the invitation to look at things differently, leaving behind the old, out-grown, painful limitations we have used to bind ourselves in suffering. And then, he welcomes you home to the effortless simplicity of yourself as you are.

Not sure where to begin? Pick up a copy of Lott's most popular book, *You're Trying Too Hard*, which strips away all the concepts that keep us searching for a greater, more spiritual, more peaceful life or self.

Made in the USA
San Bernardino, CA
13 February 2015